Blood pressure
High blood pr~
How to reduce it
without m~

Take Control of Your Blood Pressure:
Lose Weight, Feel Great and Lower
Your High Blood Pressure

Oliver Norman

Contents

Introduction

The basics of high blood pressure

The dangers of high blood pressure

Medical treatment

What you can do to control your blood pressure

Stop smoking!

Lose weight and lower your blood pressure

Eat Better

Get moving!

Reducing the sodium in your diet

Reduce your stress

Conclusion

Introduction

If you have found your way to this book, then you may have recently been diagnosed with high blood pressure or know someone that has. This condition is serious and can directly impact your overall health and life if not treated. The symptoms can go unrecognized for years and cause damage before you ever suspect that you may be suffering from them. But what exactly is high blood pressure? More importantly, once you have been diagnosed, what can you do to get them under control?

High blood pressure is a medical condition that can have serious consequences to your health. You can live with high blood pressure for years and not recognize the symptoms. high. Often the symptoms of this condition can go undetected for many years before being diagnosed because the symptoms may be subtle and easy to explain away. Although undetected, this condition can still cause severe health problems and increase your risk of heart disease, heart attack and stroke.

If you have been diagnosed with high blood pressure, your physician will prescribe a treatment plan that will help you to lower your blood pressure and decrease your chance of developing serious health issues. This book highly recommends that you follow the prescribed treatment plan that your physician has implemented for your care and treatment. That treatment plan is your best option for getting your blood pressure under control but it's not the only way.

You have full control of getting your blood pressure under control. There are so many ways that you can contribute to the success of the treatment that your doctor has prescribed for you. If you fully get on board with taking control of your blood pressure through diet and exercise you will find that not only will you get your blood pressure under control but you will also lose weight and feel great. You may even notice that you feel better than you have in years.

Through diet and exercise, you may even loose enough weight and get in great physical shape that you can reduce your high blood pressure. With a little determination and effort, you may even be able to reach a weight that is in a healthy range so that your doctor is able to reduce the amount of prescription medication that you have to take in order to control your blood pressure.

In this book, you will learn about all the ways that you can take control of your blood pressure and lose weight. You will discover how to incorporate healthy food and meal options into your life and how to begin an exercise program. You will learn how easy it is to eat better and become more active. This book will guide you as you lose weight and take control of your blood pressure.

Chapter One

The basics of high blood pressure

High blood pressure is a common medical condition that strikes many adults. It affects approximately 1 in 4 adults globally and in some areas rises to 1 in 3. High blood pressure, also known as hypertension, is a medical condition that is considered long term and has far reaching and potentially devastating consequences. Being diagnosed with high blood pressure can put you at risk for stroke, coronary artery disease, heart failure, peripheral vascular disease, chronic kidney disease and loss of vision.

This medical condition can develop over the span of many years and seem to have no symptoms or symptoms so subtle that most people are unaware that they are suffering from any form of medical ailment. Although undiagnosed, this condition can still inflict serious damage to your blood vessels and heart before it is ever detected.

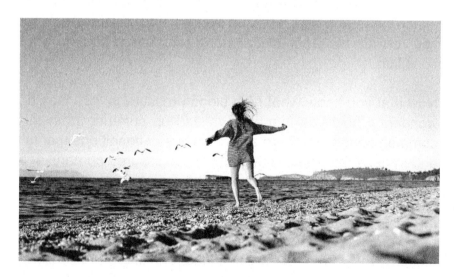

The medical condition known as high blood pressure is blood pressure in the arteritis that is consistently elevated.

Your blood pressure is actually a combination of the amount of blood that your heart pumps and the resistance to blood flow in your arteries. In the case of people that are diagnosed with high blood pressure, their heart pumps blood into arteries that have been narrowed due to many factors. The narrower your arteries the harder you heart has to work to pump blood through them. The constant force of your blood against your narrowing arterial walls is what can increase your susceptibility to other potentially life threatening ailments.

To determine if you have high blood pressure, you doctor started by measuring the systolic and diastolic pressures. Systolic pressure is the maximum pressure and normally measures from 100 to 140 millimeters mercury or mmHg. Diastolic pressure is the minimum pressure and normally measures between 60 – 90 mmHg. These numbers are normally read as systolic/diastolic. People suffering from high blood pressure have a resting systolic pressure of 140/90and higher for adults. Your blood pressure may also be measured over a 24-hour period in order to determine the exact measurements of your systolic and diastolic so that your physician can have a more accurate picture of your condition.

Now that you know what high blood pressure is, you may be wondering how you managed to end up suffering from this common condition. There are two types of conditions that fall under the blanket term high blood pressure: primary and secondary high blood pressure. The first and most common is primary high blood pressure. This condition accounts for over 90% of all cases seen in adults that suffer from high blood pressure. It is caused by habits and behaviors such as being overweight or obese, smoking, drinking and excessive sodium intake. Genetic factors may also play into your chances of developing it. as well. The second form of high blood pressure accounts for less than 10% of all case and can be attributed to an existing medical condition such as endocrine disorder or certain types of kidney disease.

If you have been diagnosed with high blood pressure, know that you are not alone. This condition affects almost everyone that you know either directly or indirectly. High blood pressure is extraordinarily common all over the world and has been dramatically increasing in developed nations over the last decades. As more people struggle with weight issues, high blood pressure will continue to rise.

Fortunately, you don't have to be one of the many people that will suffer for the rest of their lives with high blood pressure and ultimately die of an illness directly caused by their elevated blood pressure. You can choose to take control of your life, your treatment and your blood pressure. You can be in control and reduce your blood pressure.

Chapter Two

The dangers of high blood pressure

High blood pressure is a long term medical condition that can have far reaching and incredibly detrimental effects on your health and your life. The damage that this condition inflicts on the human body can cause moderate to severe issues and can make existing conditions or future conditions even more dangerous and life threatening.

The long term effects to your health from the consistent damage and stress of high blood pressure can lead to the development of coronary artery disease, also known as heart disease. This is the name of a group of conditions such angina, myocardial infarction and sudden cardiac death. It falls into the category of cardiovascular disease. Coronary artery disease is the leading cause of death in adults from around the world, accounting for nearly 1 in 5 of all deaths. Major factors that contribute to the development of this condition are high blood pressure, lack of exercise, obesity, smoking, and poor diet.

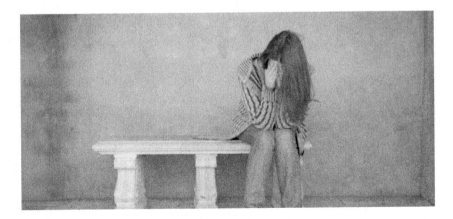

High blood pressure is the major risk factor for the development of peripheral artery disease. This condition is the narrowing of the arteries in the body which can lead to tissue death in the limbs such as the legs and amputations of affected limbs. Another major risk factor for developing this condition is high blood cholesterol which is often the result of poor diet choices. Peripheral artery disease affects over 200 million people globally each year.

Heart failure, also known as congestive heart failure is can be caused by high blood pressure and coronary artery disease, among other potential causes. Heart failure occurs when the heart is no longer to continue pumping in order to meet the body's needs. This condition affects between 2 -10 % of all adults worldwide. A person that suffers from this condition may have difficulty breathing when exercising, experience chest pain and excessive fatigue. Depending on the severity of the condition, medication and lifestyle changes may help to treat it in the moderate stages. In the severe stages, pacemakers, defibrillators and even heart transplants may be the recommended course of action.

High blood pressure is the main risk factor for stroke. A stroke is caused by either lack of blood flow to the brain or hemorrhage. A stroke is a term used to describe a cerebrovascular accident or cerebrovascular insult. High blood pressure and obesity combines can dramatically increase your chances of having a stroke. Strokes have been consistently the second leading cause of death right after coronary artery disease accounting for over 12% of all deaths globally. Strokes can be fatal and if survived can lead to paralysis, partial paralysis, reduced or greatly diminished capacity to read, speak or understand language.

High blood pressure is a contributing factor for other long term illnesses such as chronic kidney disease and loss of vision. High blood pressure can also cause sexual dysfunction and depression. Headaches, lightheadedness, vertigo, ringing in the ears, and fainting can also be caused by high blood pressure that is left untreated. Organ damage can also result from severe episodes of hypertension.

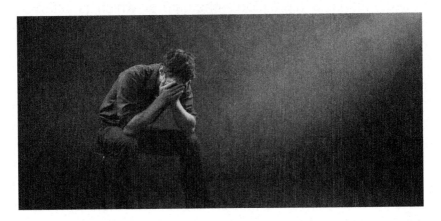

In addition, high blood pressure that stems from lifestyle choices such as poor diet, excessive drinking, smoking, obesity and lack of exercise can lead to a cycle of poor health and greatly reduced quality of life. If you are already suffering from obesity or are even overweight, make consistently poor food choices and do not exercise than you are only making your high blood pressure worse. If you suffer from high blood pressure already then you may feel tired and fatigued. This feeling of exhaustion may contribute to the lack of exercise and physical activity. You may even be tempted to eat high fat sweets and sodium rich junk food. You may consume large quantities of sodas and other beverages that are loaded with sugar and sodium. These food choices that you are consuming in order to combat your feelings of fatigue are contributing to making your high blood pressure even worse and more dangerous.

This is a vicious cycle with incredibly severe consequences. You might believe that you stuck in a loop and may feel as though you have no way out. Even though you are aware of the potentially dangerous and life threatening repercussions of the high blood pressure, you may feel depressed and powerless to make significant changes, changes that you know will lead to better health, reduce your chances of developing horrendous diseases and greatly increase the quality of your life and your overall health.

Although the tone of this chapter was serious and positively depressing at times, you do not have to accept that a diagnosis of high blood pressure from your physician spells instantaneous disaster. There are ways to treat high blood pressure. Your diagnosis does not have to be doom and gloom. Starting with your doctor's diagnosis and ending with your own determination and willingness to make changes to your lifestyle, you can take control of this condition and alter the path that you are on.

Depending on several factors such as the severity of your condition, the damage it may have already caused and your current weight and state of health, you may find that your high blood pressure is much more manageable than you thought. In the next chapter you will learn about your doctor's treatment plan and what you can do to take control of your blood pressure.

Chapter Three

Medical treatment

High blood pressure can be moderate to severe. How severe your condition is will be determined by Your physician will determine through a series of tests. Once your physician has the opportunity to assess your condition then he or she will determine the best course of action to treat your high blood pressure.

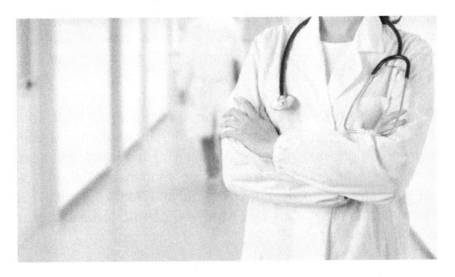

Depending in what the diagnosis may be and whether our high blood pressure falls into the moderate or severe range, you may be pleasantly surprised to find that your condition can be treated with changes in your lifestyle. A treatment plan may also include changes in diet and exercise combined with the use of medication to control your blood pressure. If you suffer from severe high blood pressure and your physician prescribed medication, then with proper use of the medication your life expectancy can be improved significantly. With proper treatment, high blood pressure can be reduced which can greatly decrease your chance of developing cardiovascular disease, heart failure, stroke and even dementia.

There are three medications that are commonly prescribed for the treatment of blood pressure. The medications account for over 90% of all medication prescribed for people that suffer from high blood pressure. These medications are in the class of drugs known as antihypertensives are used in the treatment of high blood pressure. The three most popular drugs used in treatment are thiazide diuretics, calcium channel blockers, and an ACE inhibitor. Other drugs also include angiotensin II receptor blockers, and beta blockers.

Thiazide diuretics are in the category of drugs known as diuretics which are designed to assist the kidneys rid the body of excessive amounts of sodium and water. Of all the diuretics, thiazide diuretics have consistently given the best results in people that suffer from high blood pressure and are often prescribed solely or in combination with other drugs.

Calcium channel blockers are a category of drugs that keep calcium from entering into the muscle cells of the walls of arteries, or slows the movement of calcium into the cells of the heart and blood vessels. The reduction of calcium in the cells of the blood vessels and heart improves the heart's ability to pump blood/ This category of drugs also widen the blood vessel reducing blood pressure. Calcium channel blockers can be prescribed solely or in combination with other drugs.

Angiotensin converting enzyme or ACE inhibitors are drugs often prescribed to people who are suffering form high blood pressure. This category of drugs dilates and widens the blood vessels, increases blood flow and lowers blood pressure. These drugs reduce the amount of work that the heart has to do to pump blood. ACE inhibitors are also prescribed to reduce kidney damage associated with high blood pressure.

Angiotensin II receptor blockers also known as ARBs are a category of drugs that are prescribed for the treatment of high blood pressure. These drugs cause the blood vessels to relax and widen, reducing the amount of work that the heart has to do in order to pump blood. Blood pressure is reduced when blood can flow easier through wider blood vessels. ARBs also reduce the amount of excessive sodium and water in the body by regulating the hormones which control the water and sodium balance in the body. This hormone regulation and reduction of sodium and water which also reduces blood pressure.

The category of drugs known ad beta blockers are also used in the treatment of high blood pressure. Beta Blockers are prescribed in order to lower blood pressure by reducing the amount of work that the heart has to do by disrupting the effects of the sympathetic nervous system. These drugs also help control the heart rate in people suffering from high blood pressure and have experienced accelerated heart rate.

These categories of drugs have all proven effective in the ongoing fight against high blood pressure. They are all often used singly or in a combination depending on the severity of your condition, your overall health and your physician's assessment and prognosis. These drugs can be prescribed singly or in concert with the goal of reducing your blood pressure and getting it under control.

If your doctor has proposed a regimen of these medications, then that is the treatment plan that he or she believes will get the results you are seeking and possibly even save your life. You may prefer to follow a more natural, holistic approach to dealing with your high blood pressure, but it is recommended that you at least begin your blood pressure treatment by following the sound medical advice of trained professionals.

High blood pressure is a dangerous long term medical condition that can lead to devastating medical consequences. Once diagnosed, you should do everything in your power to get it under control. There are numerous ways to approach your high blood pressure and the treatment plan can adapt to your ever changing lifestyle and to suit the present state of your condition.

Fortunately for many people that suffer from high blood pressure, the medical treatment plan is not the permanent medical solution. High blood pressure is a condition that will not force you to be on medication to control for the remainder of your life. Medical treatment may only be the beginning as you take control of your condition, but you can also make lifestyle changes and dietary changes which can have a huge impact on reducing your high blood pressure.

These changes to your lifestyle can allow you the opportunity to take control of your health and ailment. As a matter of fact, your treatment plan may include changes to your diet and activity level which may actually be prescribed by your doctor. The medical community is aware that high blood pressure is best fought with the help of many medical allies. For example, your doctor my even devise a plan that is composed of a combination of diet, exercise, stress reduction and a prescription for Thiazide diuretics.

Fortunately, if you are willing to work hard, watch what you eat, drop a few pounds and follow your doctor's advice, then you may find in only a few months' time that you have lost weight and reduced your blood pressure back into the normal range. If your doctor observes that you have lowered your blood pressure into a range that puts you well out of danger, then he or she may suggest that you no longer have to remain on the medications that he had prescribed at the onset of treatment.

If the prospect of not having to take prescription medication is not enough to motivate then think of how great you will feel when you have lost excess pounds and look great. Consider how the quality of your life can change if you only feel better about your health and have more energy. How different would your life be if you actually had the energy to do all the activities that you have dreamed about?

Chapter Four

What you can do to control your blood pressure

In the previous chapter, you learned about the different medications that are commonly prescribed to patients that have been diagnosed with high blood pressure. You discovered what the categories of drugs do and why they are prescribed. You also learned that high blood pressure can be reduced in many cases with significant changes to your lifestyle.

Depending on your condition, your doctor may suggest trying to get your blood pressure under control by making lifestyle changes before a drug regimen is prescribed, if that is the case, then your motivation will be to make sure that you do everything in your power to avoid being placed on medication.

In this chapter, you will learn about about the lifestyle changes that can have the greatest impact in reducing your high blood pressure. These changes will give you the ability iota take control of your blood pressure, lose weight and feel great! Aside from the pharmaceutical approach, there are other methods to take control of you blood pressure. Often it is a winning combination of changes made to your health, you're eating habits, and your life that will have the greatest impact to the treatment of your condition.

High blood pressure usually develops and progresses due to a number of behaviors and habits in your life. Poor diet, excessive drinking, stress, smoking, a diet filled with excess sodium, obesity, a lack of exercise all are to blame or at the very least are contributing to the diagnosis that you have received of high blood pressure. By changing these habits and improving your weight and health, you can big changes to your blood pressure and your weight.

When you are making changes to your diet, weight and lifestyle, imagine that you are reversing all the years of damage that you may have already done. If you smoke, make a commitment to stop. If you eat high fat foods and are always reaching for the salt shaker, then put the salt shaker down and order something low fat and healthy. Taking control of your blood pressure begins with you and your drive to succeed. You have to find your motivational and make the commitment to do whatever you can to lower your blood pressure.

These are the most effective ways to reduce your blood pressure:

- If you smoke, stop!
- Eat healthy and make better food choices.
- If you are overweight, lose the extra pounds.
- Limit the amount of alcohol you consume.
- Start moving and exercising.
- Find ways to reduce your stress.
- Get the rest that you need.
- Put the salt shaker down!

These topics will be covered in in detail in the next few chapters. You will learn tips and suggestions of implementing and making the necessary changes that will lead to reduced blood pressure and a better quality of life. You will discover that once you have made the commitment to your health that the ways of taking control of your high blood o pressure are simple.

With the right positive attitude, you can become more active, eat better and make a promise to yourself that you will reduce your high blood pressure. You can make the decision to begin an exercise program and shed those stubborn pounds that have been plaguing you for years. You can lose the weight and greatly reduce your chance of dealing with long term high blood pressure. You can feel great, have more energy and be confident that by following your doctor's treatment plan by doing everything that you can do to get healthier.

Chapter Five

Stop smoking!

Smoking is one of the most detrimental habits that you can develop and sustain. Not only is it a major contributing factor to the condition of high blood pressure but It contributes to cancer, heart disease, stroke, premature aging, and numerous other ailments.

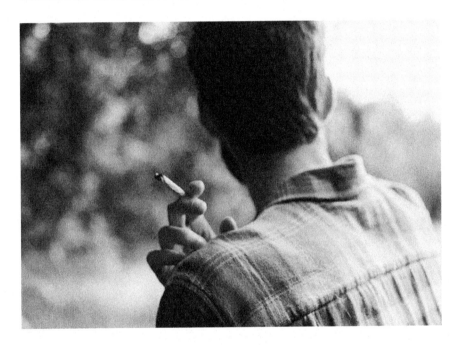

If you have developed the habit of smoking, then you may not be aware of the link between it and high blood pressure. Smoking can cause high blood pressure and increase an already developed condition. When a person smokes, smoking raises your blood pressure temporarily. It can cause damage to your arterial walls, and the chemicals found in cigarettes can damage the lining of your arteries. This damage can cause a narrowing of your arteries which leads directly to high blood pressure. Smoking can also a hardening of your arterial walls and can even lead to blood clots. Any type of smoking can cause high blood pressure; Secondhand smoke can also be a factor in the development of high blood pressure.

In the case of smoking, the best approach is to stop. Stopping smoking is not an easy task but the philosophy behind it is simple. If you are ready to take control of your blood pressure, then you will want to research the best ways and methods to stop smoking. A word of caution, any product that has nicotine in it can cause high blood pressure. if you do not smoke conventional cigarettes or are wondering if you can make the change to e-cigarettes or similar products, remember that you are still ingesting nicotine and that is causing arterial damage and high blood pressure.

When you begin to think about seriously about quitting smoking, begin to observe your habits and behaviors surrounding cigarettes. Make notes or write down your observations in a journal or notebook if it will be helpful. Make notes about how much you smoke. Ask yourself a few questions such as: what time of day do you smoke and why? What triggers you to smoke? Is it stress, social events, certain situations? Do you smoke when you are upset, nervous, angry or to relax? What is your motivation to quit smoking? Consider all these questions and write down the answers. When you decide to quit these notes will help you identify weak moments and potential pitfalls in your road to quitting smoking.

Be prepared for any potential physical and emotional side effects. Quitting smoking can be challenging and difficult at times. That is not meant to discourage you it is just meant to prepare you for the possibility that you may be facing some tough challenges at first. When you first quit smoking, you may have experience irritability, drastic mood swings, headaches, and coughing. You may be extremely hungry and crave sugar or high fat foods. You may be nauseas and not crave anything at all. You have to be prepared to give your body time to work through the stages of nicotine withdrawal.

From an emotional and mental standpoint, you may find that you are craving cigarettes almost constant. They will be foremost in your thoughts and maybe in your dreams. You may struggle to stay in control form minute to minute and then hour to hour. Just take each minute as it comes and concentrate on resisting the urge to smoke. Do whatever technique you need to do to stay in control. Your emotions may be raw and you may experience irritability. You may even notice that you have mood swings and may get easily angered. Try your best to stay focused and not let your nicotine withdrawal turn you into a monster.

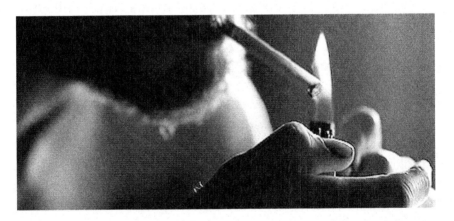

After you quit, you will find that you may struggle with the temptation to for some time. That is okay. No one is perfect and the craving for a cigarette may be something that you have to live with for a little while. Stay strong and remember that quitting smoking is an accomplishment to be proud if and it will go a long way towards helping you take control of your high blood pressure.

Follow these tips to quit smoking:

- Commit to a date. Pick a date that you will stop smoking and stick to it.
- Get rid of anything smoking related. Clear out all the cigarettes, cigars, lighters, and ashtrays out of your house and car. Do not carry anything smoking related in your purse or pockets. Clean out your desk or locker at work of anything that may tempt you to light a cigarette.
- Broadcast your decision. Talk to your doctor, tell your friends and coworkers, tell anyone that will help support you and anyone that may find themselves potentially impacted by irritability and mood swings. Your family and friends will undoubtedly be at your side and do anything they can to support you in this decision.
- Identify your smoking triggers. Do you smoke when you get stressed or at a certain time of day? Do you smoke as a reward or to relax? Once you know your smoking triggers, you can prepare to deal with them.
- Ask your doctor if patches or gum is a good solution for you.
- Find a substitute for smoking, if that is taking a deep breath, eating a piece of hard candy, sugar free gum or even low calorie foods or snacks.
- Avoid activities and places that you associate with smoking. You can return to them at some point but only after you have quit smoking for a while.
- Try to avoid people that are smoking. You do not have to give up relationships or friendships with smokers, but you may ask them not to smoke around you or choose to do something else while they are outside smoking.
- Begin an exercise program. When you smoked you probably found exercising to be hard since you may

have had difficulty breathing. Now that you have quit smoking, consider doing something fun at the gym or taking up an exercise program that you only dreamed about when you smoked.

- Cut caffeine or alcohol. If you smoked and had a cup of coffee or had a cigarette when you had an alcoholic beverage, then you may want to consider limiting these beverages for the foreseeable future.
- Reduce your stress. If you smoked to alleviate stress or in stressful situations, then find a way to diffuse stressful situations. Have a plan for long term stress relief and instant stress reduction. Breathing techniques, counting, mantras can all be used to focus your attention on something other than the source of your immediate stress. Long term stress can be managed with meditation, yoga, exercise, long walks, reading, anything that you find relaxing.
- If you find yourself craving a cigarette, concentrate on the goal that you are trying to achieve. Do you want heart disease, lung disease, or to have a stroke?
- Reward yourself. Set up rewards and milestones. Pick a time frame that means something to you. In the first weeks of quitting, reward your self frequently and often. Reward yourself for every day if it helps. Buy yourself something or earn money for every milestone you hit, such as putting money in a jar for a fabulous trip or cruise.
- Get support. Join a group in person or online. Support from people that have been there and can relate to your situation is the most empowering assistance you can get sometimes. Advice and encouragement from a nonsmoker that has been through the same struggle can mean so much when you are struggling.

Chapter Six

Lose weight and lower your blood pressure

Weight gain, being overweight and obese all contribute directly to the condition of high blood pressure. Being overweight is part of the vicious cycle that ultimately leads to and maintains high blood pressure. If you are suffering from high blood pressure, you have a reduced amount of energy, suffer from fatigue and exhaustion and are more likely to eat high fat, carbs, and sugar in order to function during the day. This diet of junk food combined with low energy level and lack of exercise leads to and maintains high blood pressure.

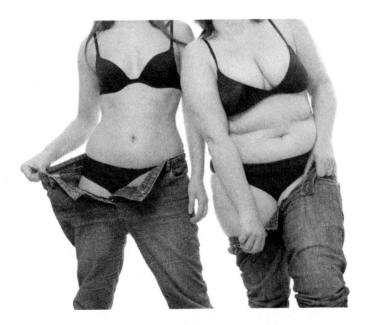

In study after study, weight loss is one of the biggest factor in lowering blood pressure. Weight loss has been proven to have a significant impact on blood pressure. The amount of weight lost does not have to be vast or in huge amounts. Even modest weight loss can reduce blood pressure from high into the normal range. If you are overweight or obese, losing weight is one of the most powerful weapons that you have in your arsenal as you take control of your blood pressure.

When a person loses weight, the number on the scale or the dress size are not all that is affected. Successfully losing weight means that you have made important changes in your diet, exercise routine and lifestyle. Heathy weight loss is almost always the result of a nutritious diet, an increase in activity, an adoption of an exercise program, and a total and complete reversal of bad habits.

If you are struggling with your weight and battling obesity than you already know what it feels like to have no energy, feel sluggish and have no motivation to exercise. You are already all too aware of how bad you feel when you wake up in the morning and at numerous times during your day. You know the fight that you have with yourself on a daily basis as you try to resist the high sugar and fatty food choices that your body craves as it drifts from one sugar crash to the next.

Being overweight isn't just about the near constant physical and mental fatigue that you feel, it is also about the way you feel about yourself and your size. You may have noticed that as your weight and blood pressure increased, your self-esteem and health decreased. This is no coincidence, there is a direct correlation between the two. Being diagnosed with high blood pressure and having extra weight are a double dose of poor health, low self-esteem, fatigue and can also be a medically dangerous combination.

One of the most important and significant changes that you can make is to lose weight. Initially, you will want to lose weight to lower blood pressure. Although you may still find after losing weight, that you are on medication to treat your condition, you may find the amount of drugs to be greatly reduced. Losing weight is a giant step toward taking control of your blood pressure.

The main motivation is to get your blood pressure under control, but you will also find that losing weight will also reduce your risk for other medical ailments such as diabetes. Losing weight will increase your self-esteem which will help you to feel better and help you to more confident. Losing weight will reduce the amount of weight that your body is forced to carry, so you may find that you now have more energy and are more motivated to exercise and be active. With more energy, you will be less likely to eat junk food to keep going. You may find that you actually enjoy a healthier, more nutritious diet when you are not eating to stay awake, conscious and focused.

The side effects and perks that you will enjoy from only losing a few pounds will be tremendous. You may even feel like a completely different person. You will be a smaller size and more confident. You will enjoy more energy and will feel much less fatigues. you will find that you do not have to rely on junk food and poor food choices just to make it through the day. You may even go through an entire day without candies, chips and junk food. Losing weight is one of most dramatic changes in lifestyle that you can do to lower your blood pressure, gain more energy and change your life.

The advantages of losing weight:

- Reduce blood pressure. This is the biggest health reason to lose weight. Obesity and high blood pressure combined are a dangerous and potentially lethal combination.
- Reduce your dependence on medication. By losing weight, you can move your blood pressure into the normal range. If you are able to sustain your weight

loss and your blood pressure in a normal range, your doctor may be able to reduce or discontinue the drug regimen that you have been placed on for your high blood pressure.

- Increase your energy. People that suffer from obesity and are overweight often develop a noticeable decrease in energy. This lack of energy affects their overall quality of life. It affects the desire to exercise and to be active, it also effects how you function during the day and whether you avoid eating junk food. By losing weight you will increase your energy and feel much better.
- Better health. Extra pounds can not only lead to high blood pressure, heart disease and increase your risk of stroke, but it can also contribute to diabetes.
- Less sick days. Being overweight and obese decreases your immune's system's ability to fight viruses and illnesses, so you spend more time sick with colds and flu.
- Live longer. Numerous studies have linked being overweight and obese to dangerous and life threatening health issues. Losing the extra pounds and attaining a healthy weight is one of the most important steps you can take in order to live a long and healthy life.
- Look better. This may seem like a superficial reason, but looking better is a great motivation to help you lose weight. Losing weight is so important that even of you lose weight just to fir into your favorite jeans, the side effects will be reduced blood pressure and better health.

The first step to losing weight is to purchase a scale. If you do not already own one, you will want to purchase a scale. The number on the scale will be reflective of fat and muscle but it will definitely give you a good idea of how much you weigh and how much you need to lose. Weigh yourself once a week. This will allow for fluctuations in water retention and due to other factors.

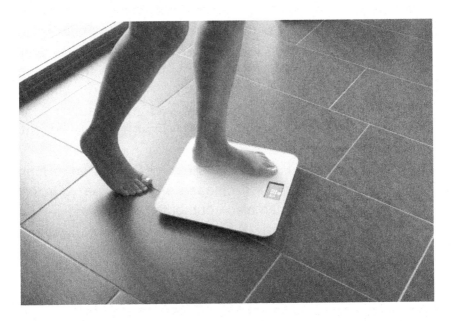

This step is hard, but necessary. Pick a day and get on the scale. Face the number staring back at you. Now that you have a starting point, you know what you need to do. Confronting that number is tough and painful but you need to know what it is so that you can change it. If you need to lose a large amount if weight, do not focus on the entire amount. Break it up into more manageable amounts. Focus on the small amounts, start with the fact that you need to lose 10 pounds, then when you achieve that goal, do 10 more pounds and so on.

Set up a reward program for your weight loss success. Set goals and decide what reward you want for achieving each goal. Rewards such as new clothes, a day at the spa, or a mini vacation will help to keep you motivated. Be sure to set up goals for small achievements and large ones. You may even consider setting a dollar mount for each pound lost and putting that amount into a jar for you to spend on your reward. The reward program that you set up will help you stay motivated.

The next step is to buy a small notebook or download an app. Find a small notebook that you can carry with you. This notebook is going to be your food diary. Write down everything you eat and drink, include the amounts, the time of day, and what you were feeling. You can even fill in the calories if you it helps to keep your diet in track. The purpose of a food diary is to help you become aware of what you are actually consuming during the day and why. Do you eat because you are stressed, bored, or angry? Do you eat mindless calories and not realize it every day? You can also download apps that will help you to keep track of calories consumed during the day.

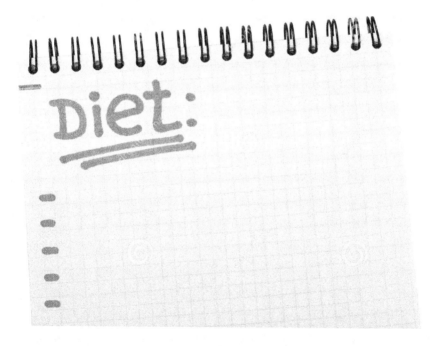

Pick a day to start your diet and broadcast it. The more people you tell the more accountable you will feel. If you are accountable to friends and family, then you are much more likely to stay on your diet and to stay motivated. You may even want to join a support group in your community or online to help you stay motivated and to share tips and successes.

Losing weight will reduce your blood pressure and help you return to a more energetic, healthier and better life. You will feel like doing more, exercising and you will spend less time sick and ill. To lose weight you will need to eat healthier and exercise. In the following chapters you will learn how to start eating better and begin a safe and healthy exercise program.

Chapter Seven

Eat Better

In the previous chapter, you learned about the importance of losing weight and the role it plays in reducing your blood pressure. To lose weight you will need to change your eating habits. You will need to rethink your approach to meals and snacks. You will need to make better food choices. In this chapter, you will learn how to eat better so that you can lose weight and reduce your blood pressure.

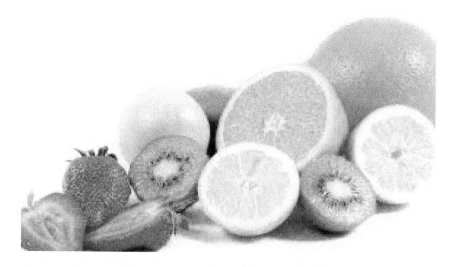

Losing weight can seem daunting but it is not impossible. You will just need to make sure tough decisions and commit to taking control of your health and blood pressure. If you stay overweight or obese, your high blood pressure can easily lead to heart disease, heart failure or stroke. At that point it may be far too late to make changes in your life. Now is the time. Make a commitment to yourself that you are going to lose weight so that you can have a long, healthy life without high blood pressure.

To lose weight, you will have to be motivated and stay motivated because every day you are going to face decisions about everything you eat. Every dish, snack, and meal will give you an opportunity to eat healthy or return to your previous bad eating habits. If you have a strategy and strong motivation, you are far more likely to be successful at losing weight. Decide what your motivation is and make a promise that you are going do your best to eat better.

The good news is that you do not have to drastically change your eating habits overnight. You can begin by making a few simple food choices that will help you to ease into a better diet. The food choices that you will make will be easy and delicious, you may not even realize that eating healthy could taste so good.

How to eat better:
- Eat more fruits and vegetables. Find ways to add fruits and vegetables into your diet. When you reach for a snack, pick a banana or apple. When you are cooking dinner, be sure to include heart heathy choices like broccoli, cauliflower, tomatoes, and dark leafy vegetables. Try to replace carbs and fatty foods with cooked vegetables or a fresh salad.
- No more fried foods. None. Fried foods are clogging your arteries and making your high blood pressure worse. Fried foods are also contributing to any weight issues that you may be experiencing. Avoid fried foods at all costs.
- No more processed cakes and sweets. Honeybuns, coffee cakes, cinnamon buns, or anything else that is cakey, sweet and loaded with fat need to be removed from your diet.

- Avoid white bread. White bread is overly processed and devoid of any real nutritional value. White bread converts easily into sugar which may be stored as fat in your body.
- Choose lean protein. Be sure that all the protein that you are consuming is lean. Do not eat skin, fat, or heavily fried products. Plant proteins are also a leaner, healthier choose than animal protein.
- Steam, boil, bake, or choose not to cook. When cooking your meals, these methods are acceptable because they do not require any oil or grease. You can steam, boil, bake or consume raw most foods and enjoy the nutrition and the taste but without the dangerous fat and extra calories.
- Avoid processed food. Processed food is anything that has chemicals, dyes, and preservatives in it. These foods are typically in the middle aisles if the grocery store. They come in boxes, bags, and packages with long shelf lives. They are usually packed with fillers, fat, and sugar.
- Drink water. Try to drink water throughout the day. Replace sweet tea, soda and any other unhealthy drink with water. Drink a glass of water before eating and anytime you feel hungry or crave something unhealthy.
- Don't skip breakfast. People that skip breakfast are more likely to overeat later in the day, so be sure to eat breakfast.
- Dinner should be light. It is far better to eat a large meal earlier in the day than later. The last meal of the day should be light since you will be going to sleep and your metabolism will be slowing down.
- Try to include whole grains. Whole grains have been proven to be healthy for your heart and for your waistline. Try to add whole grain oats, quinoa, whole wheat flour, and other similar foods into your diet.

- Use olive oil. Avoid lard, fat, butter and margarine. Try to use light and heart healthy oils such as extra virgin olive oil, coconut oil, or light vegetable oil or cooking, salads, or whenever oil or butter is called for in a recipe.
- Eat your fiber. Choose foods that are high in fiber such as fruits, vegetables, dry peas and beans. Any beans or legumes, and whole grain foods. Foods high in fiber are nutrient dense and contain vitamins and minerals.
- Pay attention to portion size. Eat only a single serving of food and be careful as to the amount of food you have n that portion. Use smaller plates and bowls to help control portion size.

Chapter Eight

Get moving!

Your high blood pressure can be reduced and controlled by a combination of losing weight and a healthy diet. Exercise is an important part of losing weight and maintaining a heathy lifestyle after you have lost all the excess pounds. Exercise and physical activity will help to control your blood pressure but also strengthen your heart. It will help you to manage your stress levels which will also help you to achieve your blood pressure goals.

Beginning an exercise program starts with a trip to your doctor's office. If you have been diagnosed with high blood pressure, you will want to consult with your doctor before beginning any physical activity. Get his or her advice since your doctor is aware of the extent and severity of your condition. Be sure that now is the right time to start moderate activity or an exercise program.

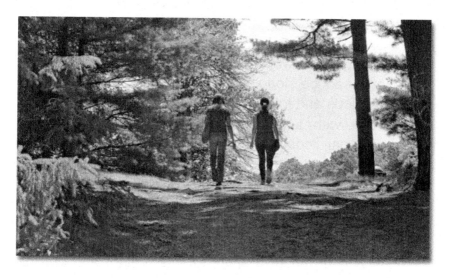

Once you have received your doctor's approval then it is time to get started. You can start an exercise program by simply walking around your neighborhood or you could join a gym. Think if exercise as fun and try to find something that appeals to you and that you will enjoy. Exercise doesn't have to drudgery or boring, it can be fun, relaxing and a great way to relieve stress. You can also add physical activity into your daily routine, get healthy, lose weight and reduce your high blood pressure.

The American Heart Association recommends at least 150 minutes of physical activity at a moderate pace per week. Since your goal is to reduce your blood pressure, then it is recommended that 3-4 times per week you engage in moderate physical activity for 40 minutes at a time. If your doctor approves it, you can engage in vigorous physical activity 40 minutes 3 – 4 times a week to improve your health and reduce your blood pressure.

These tips will help you start an exercise program and incorporate physical activity into your life:
- Go for a walk. One of the easiest ways to begin exercising, especially after any time spent sedentary is to go for a walk 3 – 4 times a week. Walking is free and can be done almost anywhere. Be sure to be cautious and follow all safety guidelines.
- Walk with a friend or pet. If your dog is in good physical condition, he would probably live to accompany you on your walks around the neighborhood. You can also go on walks with your family or friends. It's a great way to spend time catching up and exercising all at the same time.
- Swimming and water aerobics are fun! Lap swimming is one of the best ways to lose weight and get into shape. If lap swimming is too vigorous, then consider taking a water aerobics class. Water aerobics classes

are fun, low impact and great for anyone at any fitness level.

- Go for a bike ride. Do you remember how much fun you had as a child riding your bike? Well, you can do have fun like that again. With the purchase of a bike or an exercise bike at the gym, you can ride a bike and lose weight. If you purchase a bike, you can go bike riding with your friends or family and have a great time while being active.
- Sign up for an easy or moderate dance class. There are many classes to choose from at your local gym and all will help you burn calories and lose weight. Have fun!
- Mix it up! There are so many great activities that you can do, try to mix it up so you don't get bored. Mixing your exercise program and activities will also help you to work out different muscle groups and achieve a better overall level of fitness.
- Stay in the moderate range. Since you are aiming for a moderate level of intensity with any of your physical activity, try not to strain or stress yourself. During physical activity, be sure that you can talk in brief sentences while being active. If you have to stop and catch your breath tan you are probably working too hard.
- Add physical activity into your everyday life. Park farther away. If you work at a desk job, be sure to get up and walk around from time to time. Take the stairs whenever possible. Clean the house or the yard. Try to incorporate activity any way that you can during the day, this may not contribute to your exercise program but it will help you to burn more calories.
- Find fun physical activities that the whole family can do. Kayaking, hiking, mountain biking or skiing are all great activities that are fun and burn loads of calories. You can do these activities on the weekend and have

a ggrat time while you are losing weight and getting healthy.

- Reward your effort and hard work. Set goals for exercise and physical activity. Buy new running shoes or a great new work out outfit for each goal that you reach. This will keep you motivated to keep on exercising.

Beginning an exercise program starts with the desire to lose weight, get heathy and do everything you can to reduce your high blood pressure. Getting moving and exercising are great ways to reduce your blood pressure and get in great shape.

Reducing the sodium in your diet

The amount of sodium, or salt in your diet contributes to your high blood pressure. Sodium is responsible for maintaining or contributing to the condition of high blood pressure in people that suffer from the condition, and when it is reduced blood pressure levels return to normal. Reducing the sodium in your diet is an easy way to take control of your blood pressure.

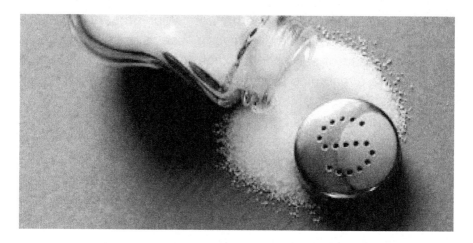

Sodium in your diet does not always come from the salt shaker. It is often found hiding in foods and beverages. Any foods or drinks that are heavily processed or contain chemicals and preservatives often have high amounts of sodium. It can also be found in foods that would seem unlikely such as salad dressing, cookies, or sweets.

One of the easiest ways to control how much sodium you are consuming on a daily basis is to limit your salt intake to less than 2.300 milligrams. Keep count of the salt consumed during the day in all foods and beverages and try not to go over that number. You may even want to keep track of your sodium intake in your food diary. Writing it down will help you to become more aware of how much salt you really do consume every day.

Reducing your salt intake does not have to be challenging, just follow these easy tips:

- Put the salt shaker down. Taste your food first before you start adding salt. Avoid putting additional salt on your food. When cooking, try not to add any more salt than necessary as you are preparing meals.
- Invest in a great collection of spices. Fresh spices and herbs are the best way to season food, but dried spice blends and herbs from your grocery store are also acceptable. You can use spices and herbs instead of salt or in addition to a little light salt. There are even spice blend combination made specifically to replace sat at the dinner table and for cooking.
- Prepare foods from scratch. When you cook foods at home, you have control over every ingredient and how much of any seasoning goes into the dish. When you are cooking food at home, you can season a dish to your tastes, so you can replace the salt with any other flavorful combination of spices, garlic, or seasoning.
- Cook foods without salt. There are so many foods that call for salt such as rice as pasta. When cooking these foods, avoid using any salt at all.
- Read food labels. Become a food detective. You will be amazed at where salt is hiding and how much. In condiments, salad dressings, desserts, cookies, salsa and hundreds more food items there is copious amounts of salt per serving. If possible to find low sodium versions of your favorite foods.
- Eat fresh or frozen whenever possible. Fresh foods and some frozen foods no sodium in them at all.

- Rinse canned food. Try to look for low sodium or no salt added versions of canned foods that you like. If there are no low sodium versions available, then be sure to rinse any canned foods thoroughly before cooking. This includes canned tuna or chicken.
- Try to avoid instant and processed foods. Instant soup, noodles, pasta based meals, soups, and any other quick, convenience food will have large amounts of sodium.

Sodium is very detrimental to your health and to your blood pressure. Try to limit your intake of sodium each day and you will soon find that your blood pressure will decrease and you will be one step closer to take control of your blood pressure.

Chapter Nine

Reduce your stress

Stress can play is a major factor in the development of high blood pressure. When you are stressed, your body produces hormones that trigger a spike in your blood pressure. This temporary spike can cause your blood vessel to become more narrow and your heart to work harder and beat at an accelerated rate. Depending on the severity of your condition additional stress can strain your heart. The hormones that are released may also cause damage to your arteries. Stress can also play a part in triggering other behaviors or habits that are detrimental to your reducing your blood pressure. Stress can act as a trigger for smoking, overeating, excessive drinking and even lack of rest.

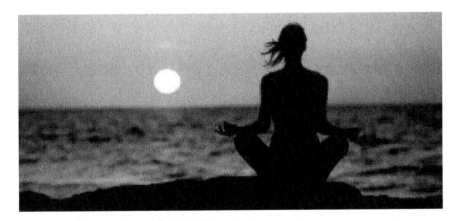

As you work to take control of your blood pressure, reducing your stress level and decreasing long term, short term and chronic stress should be part of your strategy. Reducing the amount of stress in your life and how you and your body react to stress will help you lower your blood pressure.

These are a few tips to get you started:

- Meditate. Meditation has been proven to be an effective in reducing long-term, short term, and chronic stress. Meditation can be a part of your daily routine and does not require a big time commitment to be effective. Meditating for 10 minutes or more a day a few times a week can greatly reduce your stress level, Meditation can also help you focus and react more calmly to stressful situations as they arise. There are many techniques but a simple meditation technique involves focusing I your breathing in a quiet setting.
- Take a yoga class. There are so many different types of yoga to try. Whether you choose a yoga Pilates hybrid class or prefer a more traditional d=style, yoga is very calming and is a wonderful way to reconnect with your body and reduce your stress.
- Take time to read and relax. If your schedule is a whirlwind of activity, try to find at least 30 minutes of downtime to read a book, take a hot bath and just unwind. You need this time to relive some of the tension in your life. Be sure to turn off the cell phone, television and lap top.
- Get a massage or a manicure. Try to indulge on a regular basis in a little pampering. A massage at your favorite spa or a relaxing manicure will give you a few minutes to unwind and reward yourself.
- Buy a journal and start writing. Journaling is a proven effective method of stress relief. In the pages of your journal you can write about your worries, anxieties, frustrations and joys. You can let go of the day's frustrations in your journal and get all the negativity and repressed emotions out of your system.
- Spend some time in nature. If possible take some time on a regular basis to go outside and spend time in your backyard, the park or some other green space. There is something very rejuvenating about

time spent outdoors. Take a blanket, a good book and a snack and have a picnic. Enjoy the sunshine.

- Take a class. Take a fun recreational class such as painting, creative writing, or anything else that looks interesting and fun. This is time for you to be able to relax and learn something new, so pick out anything that looks like it would be fun and relaxing.

Taking time to relax and unwind is important as you work to reduce your blood pressure. The stress in your life can cause you to stress eat, lose sleep, and have mood swings. Stress can contribute to weight issues and anxiety. By taking time to relax or find positive outlets for your stress, you can unwind and have positive, healthy outlets for your stress.

Conclusion

In this book, you learned about the dangers of high blood pressure. You discovered what high blood pressure is and the many causes of this medical condition. You learned about the many medical issues that and diseases that are caused by the damage that high blood pressure does to the body the heart and the arteries. You also learned that there were ways that you could take control of your high blood pressure.

High blood pressure has many treatment options which rely in several categories of prescription medication. Many doctors prescribe prescription medication in combinations to reduce blood pressure, flush out excess salt and water, and widen the arteries to allow for better blood flow. Although these drugs are effective, many people choose to do everything in their power to take control of their blood pressure. they do not want to have to rely on these drugs for the whole lives.

High blood pressure can often be reduced to normal levels with a little work, dedication and commitment. Losing weight, starting an exercise program, giving up smoking, eating healthier, reducing sodium and relieving stress were presented in the pages of this book for you to read, research and use to reduce your high blood pressure.

In the chapters of this book, you learned tips and suggestions to reduce your high blood pressure and reduce the amount if medication that you need to take. The impact of changes in lifestyle, diet, and activity level were explained in this book as were tried and true techniques for losing weight, feeling great and reducing high blood pressure. The goal of these methods was simple, to help you return your high blood pressure to normal and to help you lead the best, healthiest and longest life possible.

By taking control of your blood pressure, you can improve your health and live your life to the fullest. You will look better, feel great, and live a life unencumbered by the side effects and long term health issues if high blood pressure. By taking control of you blood pressure, you can now life your life the way you want to and on your terms. You don't have to let high blood pressure control of your life, you have the power to take control of your blood pressure and your health.

It is time to take control of your blood pressure, lose weight, feel great and lower your blood pressure!

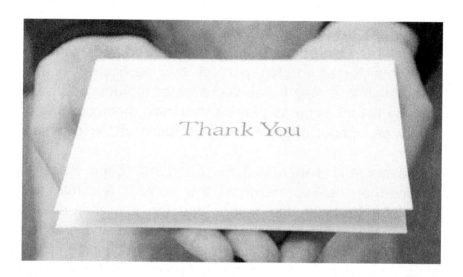

If you enjoyed this book and found it helpful and informative, please leave a positive review. Thank you.